YOGA FOR STRESS RELIEF

Embrace Yoga for Stress-Free Living

Steven m. Bowman

Table of contents

Introduction

Stress has become an all-too-common companion in our lives in today's fast-paced society.

The demands of work, relationships, and the ever-increasing pace of technology can leave us feeling overwhelmed and drained. But fear not, for within the pages of this book, we embark on a journey towards a simpler, calmer, and more centered you through the practice of yoga.

Why Yoga for Stress Relief?

Yoga offers a time-tested and holistic approach to managing stress. It's not about contorting your body into impossible positions or becoming a human pretzel. Instead, it's a gentle, accessible, and empowering way to reconnect with your inner self, find peace amidst chaos, and restore balance to your life.

Benefits of Practising Yoga

By the end of this book, you'll discover how yoga can help you reduce stress and anxiety, improve your physical and mental well-being, and cultivate a sense of inner harmony. You don't need to be flexible, fit, or spiritually enlightened to start; all you need is an open mind and a willingness to embark on this journey with us.

Who This Book Is For

This book is for anyone who seeks a respite from the relentless pressures of modern life. Whether you're a stressed-out student, a busy professional, a parent juggling multiple responsibilities, or simply someone looking for a way to bring more tranquillity into your world, this book is your roadmap to a calmer existence.

How to Use This Book

We've designed this book with simplicity and your needs in mind. Each chapter is structured to provide easy-to-follow guidance, from understanding the basics of yoga to practical yoga poses and mindfulness techniques. You can read it cover to cover or jump directly to the sections that resonate with you the most.

Throughout these pages, you'll find practical advice, clear explanations, and simple exercises that you can incorporate into your daily life. The aim is to make yoga for stress relief accessible, enjoyable, and transformative.

So, let's embark on this journey together. Take a deep breath, open your heart, and step onto the path of yoga for stress relief. It's a journey that promises not just relaxation but also self-discovery, resilience, and a life with more serenity. Welcome aboard!

Chapter 1: Understanding Stress

What Is Stress?

Stress is a part of our daily lives, and chances are, you've felt its effects more times than you can count. But what exactly is stress? At its core, stress is your body's natural response to any demand or threat. It's the "fight or flight" mechanism that has evolved over thousands of years to help us survive.

In simpler terms, when faced with a challenging situation, your body releases stress hormones like cortisol and adrenaline. These hormones prepare you to either confront the threat or run from it. Your heart rate increases, your muscles tense up, and your senses become sharper. This response is designed to be a temporary burst of energy to help you deal with immediate danger.

Different Types of Stress

Stress isn't a one-size-fits-all experience. There are different types of stress, and it's important to recognize them:

Acute Stress: This is the most common form of stress and usually occurs in response to everyday pressures and challenges. It's the tension you feel before a presentation, an important exam, or a job interview.

Chronic Stress: Chronic stress is long-term and often stems from ongoing issues such as work-related stress, financial problems, or relationship difficulties. It can wear you down over time and lead to physical and emotional health problems.

Episodic Acute Stress: Some people seem to live in a constant state of acute stress. They jump from one crisis to another, and this can take a toll on their well-being.

Traumatic Stress: This type of stress results from exposure to traumatic events like accidents, natural disasters, or violence. On mental health, it may have long-lasting consequences.

The Impact of Stress on Your Health

Understanding the impact of stress on your health is crucial. When stress becomes chronic or overwhelming, it can affect your body and mind in various ways:

Physical Health: Chronic stress has been linked to a range of health issues, including heart disease, high blood pressure, digestive problems, and a weakened immune system.

Mental Health: Stress can contribute to anxiety, depression, and other mental health disorders. It can also impair cognitive function and memory.

Behavioural Changes: Stress often leads to unhealthy coping mechanisms such as overeating, excessive alcohol consumption, or smoking.

Relationship Strain: Stress can strain relationships, leading to conflict and a decreased quality of life.

As we delve deeper into the practice of yoga for stress relief, remember that understanding stress is the first step toward managing it effectively. The techniques and practices you'll learn in this book will help you build resilience, regain control over your body and mind, and ultimately lead a more peaceful and balanced life.

Chapter 2: Getting Started with Yoga

What Is Yoga?

Yoga is a voyage of self-discovery and wellbeing, not merely a physical workout.

At its core, yoga is a holistic practice that unites your mind, body, and spirit. It's about finding balance, both within yourself and in relation to the world around you.

Preparing for Your Yoga Practice

Before you dive into yoga, it's important to make a few preparations:

Wear comfortable, loose-fitting attire that doesn't restrict your movement.

You don't need designer yoga outfits; any attire that lets you stretch comfortably will do.

Quiet Space: Find a quiet space where you won't be easily distracted. It could be a corner of your living room, a park, or even your backyard. Creating a peaceful environment can enhance your yoga experience.

Yoga Mat: While not mandatory, a yoga mat provides a stable and comfortable surface for your practice.

If you don't have one, a non-slippery surface like a carpet or a rug will work.

Time Commitment: Decide how much time you can dedicate to your practice. Starting with just 10-15 minutes a day is perfectly fine. Consistency matters more than the duration.

Finding the Right Environment

Creating the right environment for your yoga practice can significantly impact your experience. Here are some tips:

Natural Light: If possible, practice in natural light. It can uplift your mood and help you feel more connected to the world around you.

Clean Space: Ensure your practice area is clean and clutter-free. A neat environment might aid with mental clarity.

Quietude: Choose a time when your environment is relatively quiet. Silence or soothing background music can enhance your focus.

Basic Yoga Equipment

Yoga doesn't require a lot of fancy equipment. Here are some basic items you might find useful:

Yoga Mat: As mentioned earlier, a yoga mat provides a comfortable surface and better grip.

Yoga Blocks: These foam or wooden blocks can assist you in poses if you're not very flexible. They're great for beginners.

Yoga Strap: A strap can help you reach your toes or hold stretches more comfortably.

Blanket: A blanket can be used as cushioning or to cover yourself during relaxation poses.

Remember, yoga is about simplicity and self-discovery. You don't need to rush into complex poses or buy expensive gear. It's a personal journey, and the most important thing is to start and gradually build your practice. In the following chapters, we'll explore gentle yoga poses, breathing techniques, and meditation practices to help you find stress relief, balance, and tranquillity in your life.

Chapter 3: Yoga Poses for Stress Relief

In this chapter, we'll explore a variety of gentle yoga poses that are designed to melt away stress and tension from your body and mind. Remember, you don't need to be a seasoned yogi to benefit from these poses. They are accessible to beginners and can be adapted to your comfort level.

Gentle Yoga Poses

Child's Pose (Balasana): Begin your practice with this comforting pose. Kneel on the floor, sit back on your heels, and stretch your arms forward while lowering your forehead to the ground. This posture helps you connect with your breath and provides a gentle stretch for your back.

Cat-Cow Stretch: On your hands and knees, alternate between arching your back (cow) and rounding it (cat). This flowing movement warms up your spine and releases tension in the back and neck.

Downward-Facing Dog (Adho Mukha Svanasana): This classic yoga pose stretches your entire body. Starting on your hands and knees, pull your hips upward into the shape of an inverted V.It's excellent for releasing tension in the shoulders and hamstrings.

Standing Forward Bend (Uttanasana): Stand with your feet hip-width apart and bend forward, reaching for your toes. This pose is great for stretching the entire back of your body and calming the mind.

Legs-Up-The-Wall Pose (Viparita Karani): Lie on your back with your legs extended upward against a wall. This pose promotes relaxation and helps reduce swelling in the legs and feet.

Yoga Breathing Techniques

Breathing is a fundamental aspect of yoga for stress relief. Here are two simple techniques to get you started:

Deep Belly Breathing: Sit or lie down comfortably, place one hand on your chest and the other on your abdomen. Expand your diaphragm by taking a deep breath in through your nose, then gently let it out through your mouth.

This breath calms your nervous system.

4-7-8 Breath: Inhale quietly through your nose for a count of four, hold your breath for a count of seven, and exhale completely through your mouth for a count of eight. This technique helps regulate your breath and reduce anxiety.

Mindful Meditation

Meditation is a powerful tool for stress reduction. Start with short sessions and gradually extend your practice. Sit down in a comfortable posture, close your eyes, and concentrate on your breathing. Bring your focus back to your breath when it naturally wanders (which it will). Meditation helps clear mental clutter and brings calmness to your thoughts.

Creating a Relaxing Routine

As you explore these yoga poses, breathing techniques, and meditation practices, consider incorporating them into a daily routine. Consistency is key to experiencing the full benefits of yoga for stress relief. In the next chapters, we'll delve deeper into specific poses and techniques to help you build a comprehensive stress-relief practice that fits seamlessly into your life.

Chapter 4: Yoga for Physical Relaxation

In this chapter, we'll explore specific yoga poses and techniques aimed at releasing physical tension from various parts of your body. These poses can be especially helpful for those who carry stress in their muscles and want to experience physical relaxation.

Neck and Shoulder Tension Release

Neck Rolls: Sit comfortably or stand with your feet shoulder-width apart. Gently drop your head to one side and roll it in a circular motion, then switch directions. This helps alleviate tension in the neck and shoulders.

Eagle Arms: Cross your right arm over your left and bring your palms together if possible. Lift your elbows to shoulder height, and if you can, hook your right elbow over the left. The upper back and shoulders are the focus of this stretch.

Back and Spine Relaxation

Cat-Cow Stretch (Continued): This pose, mentioned earlier, deserves another mention. The rhythmic arching and rounding of your spine helps to relieve tension and stiffness in your back.

Child's Pose (Variation): Extend your arms forward in Child's Pose to gently stretch your spine. This variation can help release tension in the lower back.

Hip and Lower Body Stretches

Butterfly Pose (Baddha Konasana): Sit with the soles of your feet together and your knees bent outward.Gently push your knees while holding your feet. toward the floor. This pose eases tension in the hips and groyne.

Seated Forward Bend (Paschimottanasana): Sit with your legs extended and hinge at your hips to reach for your toes. The lower back and hamstrings are the focus of this stretch.

Yoga for Better Sleep

Supine Spinal Twist: Lie on your back, bend your knees, and drop them to one side while keeping your shoulders on the ground. This twist relaxes the spine and can promote better sleep.

Legs-Up-The-Wall Pose (Continued): This pose, mentioned in Chapter 3, is excellent for reducing leg and lower back tension. It can be especially helpful for those dealing with restless legs or insomnia.

By incorporating these poses into your yoga practice, you'll gradually release physical tension and stiffness. Remember, it's essential to practice patience and listen to your body. Push yourself gently, but never to the point of pain. In the next chapter, we'll explore yoga practices specifically designed to calm the mind and provide mental relaxation, complementing the physical relaxation techniques you've learned here.

Chapter 5: Yoga for Mental Calmness

In this chapter, we'll delve into yoga practices and techniques designed to calm your mind, reduce stress, and promote mental tranquility. These exercises will help you find balance and inner peace amidst life's challenges.

Mind-Body Connection

Before we dive into specific yoga practices, it's important to understand the mind-body connection in yoga. Yoga encourages you to pay attention to the sensations in your body as you move through poses and focus on your breath. This mindfulness fosters a deep connection between your physical and mental states, promoting relaxation and awareness.

Stress-Reducing Yoga Asanas

Seated Meditation: Begin your practice with a few minutes of seated meditation. Find a place that is peaceful, sit down, close your eyes, and concentrate on your breathing.This simple practice calms the mind and prepares you for deeper relaxation.

Mountain Pose (Tadasana): Stand tall with your feet hip-width apart and your arms by your sides. This foundational pose promotes grounding and balance, helping you centre your thoughts.

Warrior II (Virabhadrasana II): This strong pose encourages strength and focus. It's a great way to build mental resilience as you hold the posture and direct your gaze forward.

Corpse Pose (Savasana): Lie flat on your back with your arms by your sides and your palms facing up. Close your eyes and relax completely. Savasana is a pose of deep relaxation and is often considered one of the most important parts of a yoga practice.

Yoga Nidra for Deep Relaxation

Yoga Nidra, or yogic sleep, is a guided meditation technique that induces a state of deep relaxation while maintaining awareness. It's particularly effective for reducing stress and anxiety.

During a Yoga Nidra session, you'll be guided to focus on different parts of your body, your breath, and positive affirmations. This practice can be a powerful tool to release mental tension and promote a sense of calmness.

Cultivating Mindfulness

Mindfulness is a key component of yoga for mental calmness. **It entails living in the moment fully and without holding anything back.** You can practise mindfulness during your yoga sessions and also apply it to your everyday life.

Breath Awareness: Pay attention to your breath as you move through yoga poses. Deep, mindful breathing helps you stay connected to the present moment.

Mindful Eating: Apply mindfulness to your meals by savouring each bite, eating slowly, and paying attention to the flavours and textures of your food.

Daily Mindfulness Practice: Set aside a few minutes each day for mindfulness meditation. This can help you manage stress more effectively.

As you explore these practices, remember that yoga is a journey, not a destination. It's about progress, not perfection. Consistency and patience are your allies on this path to mental calmness and inner peace. In the next chapter, we'll explore the connection between nutrition and stress and how your diet can play a role in managing stress effectively.

Chapter 6: Nutrition and Stress

In this chapter, we'll explore the essential connection between what you eat and how it impacts your stress levels. You'll discover how making mindful choices in your diet can significantly influence your ability to manage stress effectively.

The Link Between Diet and Stress

It may surprise you to learn that the food you consume has a direct impact on your stress levels. What you eat can either exacerbate stress or help you build resilience to it. Here's how:

Stress Hormones: Certain foods, especially those high in sugar and processed ingredients, can lead to spikes and crashes in blood sugar levels. These fluctuations can trigger the release of stress hormones, leaving you feeling more anxious and irritable.

Nutrient Deficiencies: A poor diet can lead to nutrient deficiencies, which can affect your mental health. For example, low levels of vitamins and minerals like B vitamins, magnesium, and omega-3 fatty acids have been linked to increased stress and mood disorders.

Gut-Brain Connection: There's a strong connection between your gut and your brain. The gut microbiome, composed of trillions of microorganisms, plays a significant role in regulating mood and stress. A healthy diet supports a balanced gut microbiome.

Stress-Reducing Foods

Here are some things to include in your diet that can help you feel less stressed:

Complex Carbohydrates: Foods like whole grains, sweet potatoes, and brown rice provide a steady release of energy and can help stabilise blood sugar levels.

Lean Proteins: Include lean proteins in your meals, such as chicken, fish, tofu, and beans They contain amino acids that are essential for the production of neurotransmitters related to mood regulation.

Fruits and Vegetables: A colourful array of fruits and vegetables provides a wide range of vitamins, minerals, and antioxidants that support overall well-being.

Nuts and Seeds: These are excellent sources of healthy fats and magnesium, which can help reduce stress and anxiety.

Yoga-Friendly Recipes

Incorporate these stress-reducing foods into your diet with some delicious, yoga-friendly recipes, such as:

Mediterranean Quinoa Salad: Packed with whole grains, colourful vegetables, and olive oil, this salad is not only nutritious but also bursting with flavour.

Green Smoothie: Blend spinach, banana, almond milk, and a tablespoon of flaxseeds for a nutrient-rich, stress-busting smoothie.

Herbal Teas: Replace your usual caffeine with calming herbal teas like chamomile or lavender.

By making thoughtful choices in your diet and incorporating stress-reducing foods, you can support your body's ability to cope with stress. Remember that your nutrition is an essential part of your overall well-being, complementing the physical and mental relaxation techniques you've learned in earlier chapters.

In the next chapter, we'll explore how to integrate yoga into your everyday life, whether you're at work, at home, or facing challenging situations, to effectively manage stress in real-world scenarios

Chapter 7: Yoga for Everyday Life

In this chapter, we'll explore how to seamlessly integrate yoga into your daily routine, whether you're at work, at home, or facing challenging situations. By applying yoga principles to real-world scenarios, you can effectively manage stress and maintain a sense of calm in your everyday life.

Yoga for Stress at Work

Desk Yoga: Incorporate short yoga stretches and breathing exercises at your desk. Simple moves like neck rolls, shoulder shrugs, and deep breaths can relieve tension during a busy workday.

Mindful Breaks: Take quick breaks to leave your work area. Use this time for mindful walking, deep breathing, or a quick seated meditation to reset your focus and reduce stress.

Chair Yoga: Explore chair yoga poses that can be done while sitting. These poses can alleviate the physical strain of sitting for extended periods and help you stay energised.

Yoga for Stress in Relationships

Couples Yoga: Practising yoga with your partner can strengthen your connection. Try partner yoga poses that encourage trust and communication.

Mindful Communication: Apply yoga principles of presence and mindfulness to your conversations. Listen actively, speak with kindness, and pause before reacting during disagreements.

Breath Control: In moments of stress or anxiety, return to your breath. Practise deep, calming breaths to centre yourself and make more thoughtful decisions.

Yoga on-the-Go: Carry your yoga practice with you. Use travel time for seated stretches or mindfulness exercises. Yoga can be practised anywhere, making it a valuable tool for stress relief when you're on the move.

Emergency Relaxation: Create a mental "emergency relaxation toolkit." This may include quick visualisation exercises or mantra repetition to calm your mind during high-pressure situations.

Remember, yoga isn't confined to a studio or mat; it's a way of approaching life with mindfulness and balance. By incorporating these practices into your everyday life, you'll build resilience to stress and improve your overall well-being.

In the next chapter, we'll explore strategies for building a sustainable yoga practice. You'll learn how to set realistic goals, stay consistent, track your progress, and adapt your practice over time to continue reaping the benefits of yoga for stress relief.

Chapter 8: Building a Sustainable Practice

In this chapter, we'll explore strategies for not only starting your yoga journey but also sustaining it over the long term. A consistent yoga practice is key to experiencing lasting benefits for stress relief and overall well-being.

Setting Realistic Goals

Define Your Intentions: Start by clarifying why you want to practise yoga. Is it for stress relief, improved flexibility, or mental clarity? You may set meaningful goals by being aware of your reasons.

Start Small: Begin with achievable goals. If you're new to yoga, commit to practising for just a few minutes each day or a couple of times a week. Gradually increase your practice duration as you become more comfortable.

Be Specific: Make your goals specific and measurable. Instead of saying, "I want to reduce stress," try, "I aim to practise yoga for 15 minutes every morning to reduce stress."

Staying Consistent

Create a Routine: Incorporate yoga into your daily or weekly routine. Consistency is key to building a lasting practice. Set aside dedicated time for yoga, just like you would for any other activity.

Use Reminders: Set alarms or reminders on your phone or calendar to nudge you to practise. It will eventually turn into a habit

Find an Accountability Partner: Practice with a friend or join a yoga class to stay motivated. Knowing that someone else is expecting you can be a powerful incentive to stay consistent.

Tracking Your Progress

Keep a Yoga Journal: Maintain a journal to record your yoga sessions, thoughts, and how you feel before and after practice. This allows you to track your progress and reflect on your journey.

Recognise and enjoy your accomplishments, no matter how modest they may be. Each step forward is a victory on your path to stress relief and well-being.

Adapting Your Practice Over Time

Pay attention to your body's messages by keeping an ear to the ground. If you feel fatigued or sore, it's okay to take a gentler practice or a rest day. Yoga emphasises respecting your body's demands.

Explore Different Styles: Experiment with various yoga styles to keep your practice fresh and enjoyable. There are many forms of yoga, from restorative to power yoga, to suit different preferences and goals.

Set New Goals: As you progress, revisit your goals and set new ones. This keeps your practice engaging and helps you continue to grow both physically and mentally.

Building a sustainable yoga practice is not about perfection; it's about commitment, flexibility, and self-compassion. Over time, you'll find that yoga becomes a natural part of your life, offering you a sanctuary of calm and balance amidst the demands of everyday living.

In the final chapter, we'll wrap up our journey, summarizing the key takeaways and providing additional resources to support your ongoing practice of yoga for stress relief.

Conclusion: The Journey Ahead

As we conclude our exploration of "Yoga for Stress Relief," it's important to reflect on the journey you've embarked upon and the transformative potential it holds for your life.

A Life with Less Stress

Throughout this book, you've discovered that yoga is not merely a physical practice but a holistic approach to achieving balance and harmony in your life. It offers you a sanctuary where you can find relief from the pressures of the modern world.

By practising yoga for stress relief, you've learned how to:

Understand stress and its various forms.

Use yoga poses, breathing techniques, and meditation to release physical and mental tension.

Make mindful dietary choices to support your well-being.

Integrate yoga into your daily life, even in challenging situations.

Your Yoga for Stress Relief Toolkit

You now possess a toolkit filled with practical exercises, breathing techniques, yoga poses, and mindfulness practices. These tools are yours to use whenever you need them, providing a path to inner peace and resilience in the face of life's challenges.

The Journey Continues

Your journey with yoga is not limited to the pages of this book. It's a lifelong exploration of self-discovery and well-being. As you continue your practice, keep in mind:

Embrace Progress, Not Perfection: Your yoga journey is unique, and it's perfectly okay to have good days and not-so-good days. Each step forward, no matter how small, is progress.

Nurture Self-Compassion: Be kind to yourself. Yoga is not about achieving impossible poses; it's about the journey, the process, and the self-love that accompanies it.

Explore and Evolve: The world of yoga is vast and diverse. Continue to explore different styles, techniques, and approaches to find what resonates most with you.

Additional Resources

To support your ongoing yoga journey, here are some additional resources:

Yoga studios and local classes in your area.

Online yoga videos and tutorials for at-home practice.

Books and publications on yoga philosophy, anatomy, and advanced techniques.

Yoga communities and forums for connecting with like-minded practitioners.

Final Words

As you move forward, remember that yoga is a lifelong practice that adapts and grows with you. It's a path toward self-discovery, inner peace, and a life with less stress. Embrace it with an open heart and an open mind, and let it guide you on a journey to a more balanced, harmonious, and stress-free life.

Thank you for joining us on this journey. May your yoga practice continue to bring you clarity, tranquillity, and lasting well-being. Namaste.

Appendix: Resources for Your Yoga Journey

In this appendix, you'll find a collection of valuable resources to enhance your understanding of yoga, deepen your practice, and find support on your journey to stress relief and well-being.

Frequently Asked Questions

What should I wear for yoga practice?

Wear comfortable, breathable clothing that allows for free movement. Avoid clothing that restricts your range of motion.

How frequently should I do yoga to decompress?

Consistency is more important than frequency. Start with a few minutes each day or a few times a week and gradually increase as you become more comfortable.

Can I do yoga if I'm not flexible?

Absolutely! Yoga is for everyone, regardless of flexibility. Many poses can be modified to suit your level of flexibility and comfort.

Is it necessary to meditate during yoga practice?

Meditation is an integral part of yoga, but it's not mandatory. You can choose to incorporate meditation or simply focus on the physical aspects of yoga if you prefer.

Yoga Glossary

A concise glossary of commonly used yoga terms and their meanings to help you understand yoga terminology.

Recommended Reading

A list of books that delve deeper into various aspects of yoga, including philosophy, practice, anatomy, and meditation. These resources can give you helpful advice and insights:

T.K.V. Desikachar's "The Heart of Yoga: Developing a Personal Practise"

"Light on Yoga" by B.K.S. Iyengar The Key Muscles of Yoga" by Ray Long "The Miracle of Mindfulness" by Thich Nhat Hanh" The Joy of Living: Unlocking the Secret and Science of Happiness" by Yongey Mingyur Rinpoche

Additional Online Resources

Explore the vast world of online resources, including websites, forums, and videos, to further enrich your yoga journey:

Yoga Journal (www.yogajournal.com): A comprehensive source of articles, poses, and practice tips.

Yoga Alliance (www.yoga alliance.org): Provides information about certified yoga teachers and studios.

Yoga With Adriene (www.yoga with adriene.com): Offers free yoga videos for practitioners of all levels.

r/yoga on Reddit (www.reddit.com/r/yoga): A community of yoga enthusiasts sharing advice and experiences.

These resources can help you expand your knowledge, find inspiration, and connect with the global yoga community.

As you continue your yoga journey, remember that learning and growth are ongoing processes. Investigate, try things out, and see what works best for you. Yoga has the potential to bring lasting peace, balance, and stress relief into your life. May your path be filled with serenity and self-discovery. Namaste.

Yoga journal

How to use this Journal

Here's a guide on how you can use this Simple Daily Journal

- Date: Start each entry with the date, allowing you to track your entries and organize them chronologically.

- Title or Heading: Consider adding a brief title or heading to each entry to summarize the main focus or theme of the day's journaling.

- Mood or Emotion Tracker: You might want to include a section or section heading to record your current mood or emotions. You can use a scale (e.g., 1-5) or descriptive terms (e.g., happy, sad, excited) to capture how you're feeling.

- Things that I am grateful for: Consider adding a dedicated space to express things you're grateful for each day. Gratitude journaling can have numerous positive effects on well-being.

- Goals and Intentions: Include a section where you can write down your goals, intentions, or affirmations for the day or the future. This helps with focus and motivation.

- Reflections: Add a section where you can reflect on the events of the day, any insights you gained, or lessons learned.

- What I accomplished today: Dedicate a spot to celebrate your accomplishments or positive things you've done during the day, no matter how big or small.

- Space for Creativity: If you enjoy creative expression, you can add an area for doodling, sketches, or any form of art that complements your journaling.

Daily Journal

Title: ________________________   Date: __________

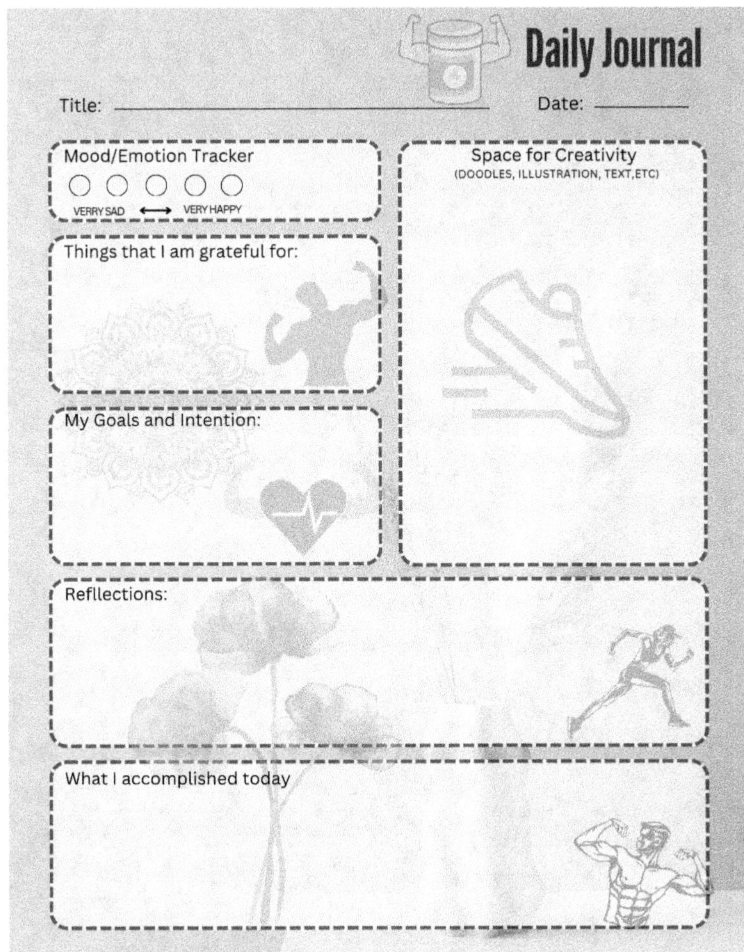

Mood/Emotion Tracker

○ ○ ○ ○ ○

VERRY SAD ←→ VERY HAPPY

Things that I am grateful for:

My Goals and Intention:

Space for Creativity
(DOODLES, ILLUSTRATION, TEXT,ETC)

Refllections:

What I accomplished today

Daily Journal

Title: ___________________________   Date: ___________

Mood/Emotion Tracker

○ ○ ○ ○ ○

VERRY SAD ←——→ VERY HAPPY

Things that I am grateful for:

My Goals and Intention:

Space for Creativity
(DOODLES, ILLUSTRATION, TEXT,ETC)

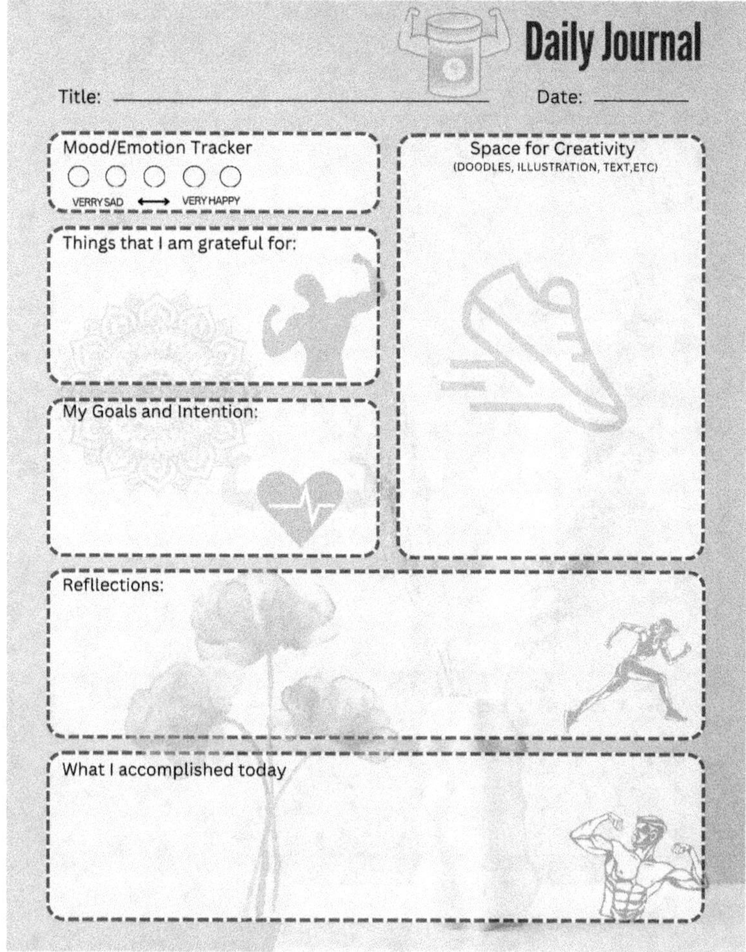

Refllections:

What I accomplished today

Daily Journal

Title: ________________________ Date: ________

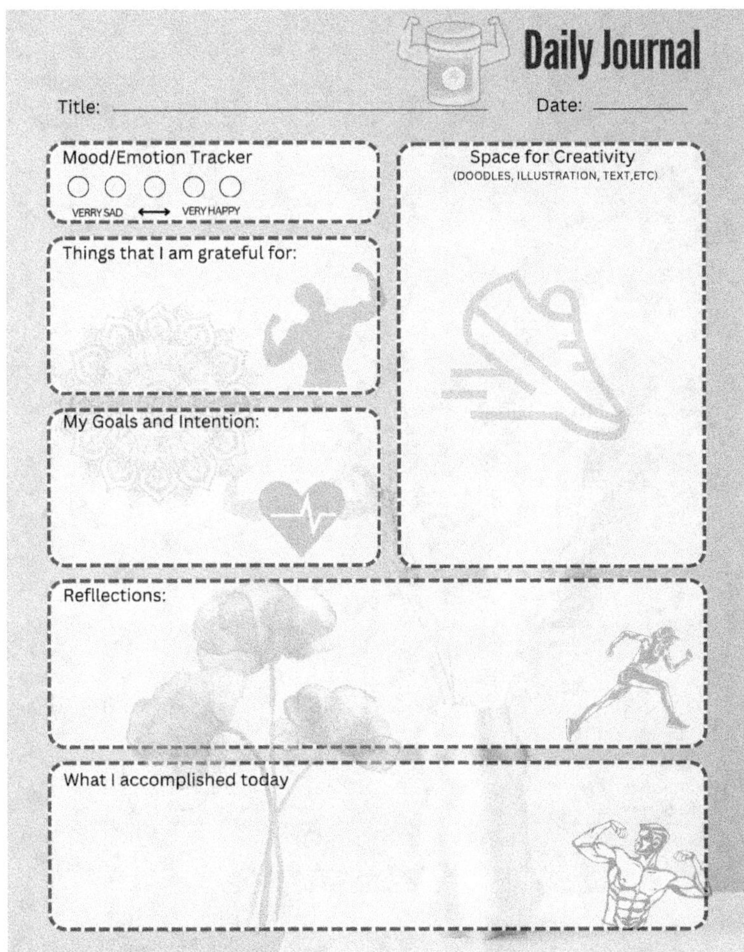

Mood/Emotion Tracker

○ ○ ○ ○ ○

VERRY SAD ←→ VERY HAPPY

Things that I am grateful for:

My Goals and Intention:

Space for Creativity
(DOODLES, ILLUSTRATION, TEXT,ETC)

Refllections:

What I accomplished today

Daily Journal

Title: ______________________________   Date: __________

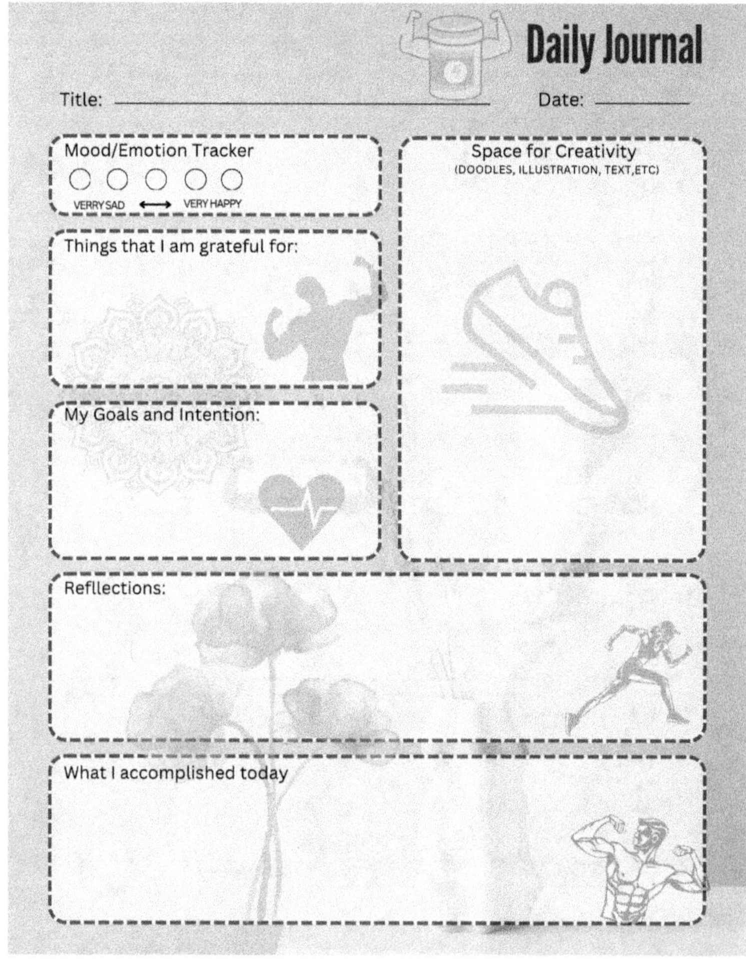

Mood/Emotion Tracker

○ ○ ○ ○ ○

VERRY SAD ←——→ VERY HAPPY

Things that I am grateful for:

My Goals and Intention:

Space for Creativity
(DOODLES, ILLUSTRATION, TEXT,ETC)

Refllections:

What I accomplished today

Daily Journal

Title: ___________________________   Date: ___________

Mood/Emotion Tracker

○ ○ ○ ○ ○

VERRY SAD ⟷ VERY HAPPY

Things that I am grateful for:

My Goals and Intention:

Space for Creativity
(DOODLES, ILLUSTRATION, TEXT,ETC)

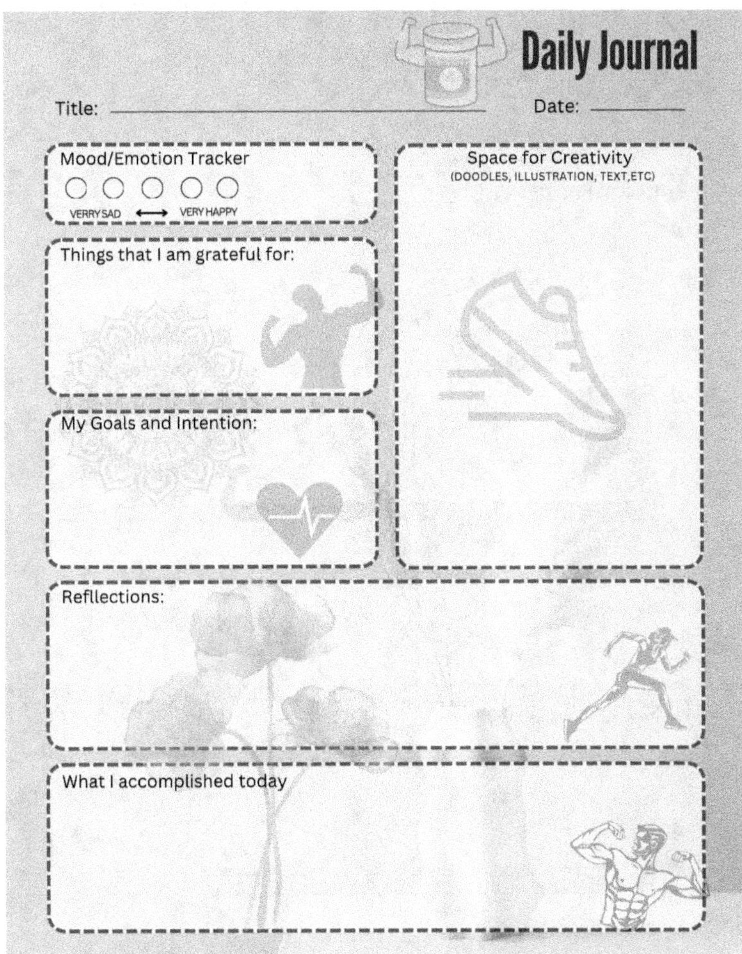

Refllections:

What I accomplished today

Daily Journal

Title: ___________________________   Date: _________

Mood/Emotion Tracker

○ ○ ○ ○ ○

VERRY SAD ⟷ VERY HAPPY

Things that I am grateful for:

My Goals and Intention:

Space for Creativity
(DOODLES, ILLUSTRATION, TEXT,ETC)

Refllections:

What I accomplished today

Daily Journal

Title: _______________________   Date: _______

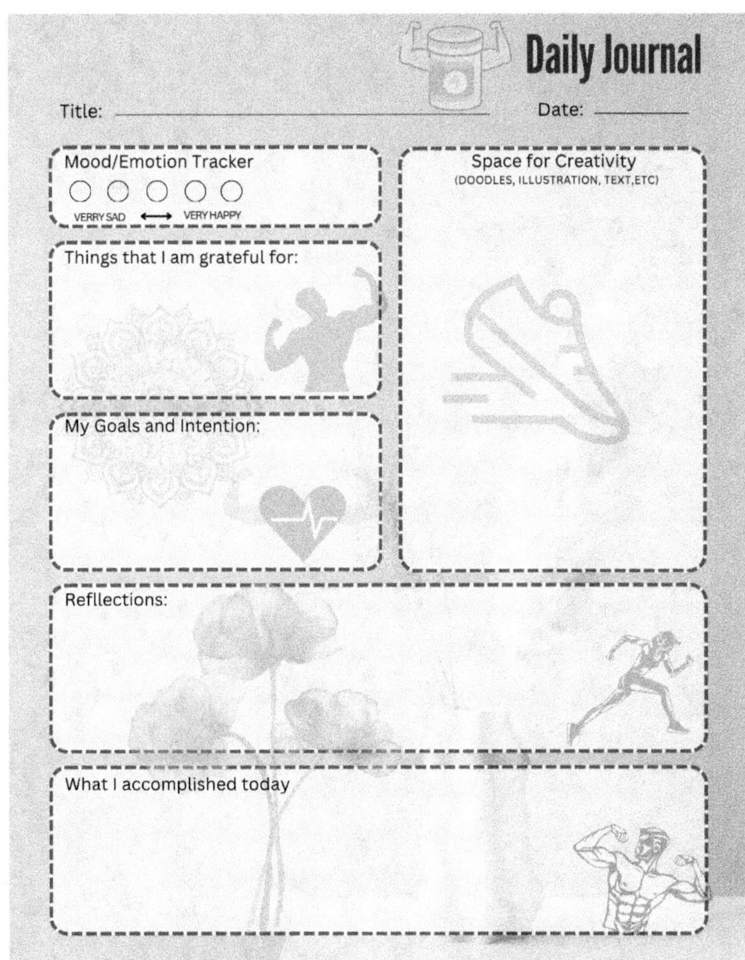

Mood/Emotion Tracker

○ ○ ○ ○ ○

VERRY SAD ⟷ VERY HAPPY

Things that I am grateful for:

My Goals and Intention:

Space for Creativity
(DOODLES, ILLUSTRATION, TEXT,ETC)

Refllections:

What I accomplished today

Daily Journal

Title: _______________________________   Date: _________

Mood/Emotion Tracker

○ ○ ○ ○ ○

VERRY SAD ⟷ VERY HAPPY

Things that I am grateful for:

My Goals and Intention:

Refllections:

What I accomplished today

Space for Creativity
(DOODLES, ILLUSTRATION, TEXT,ETC)

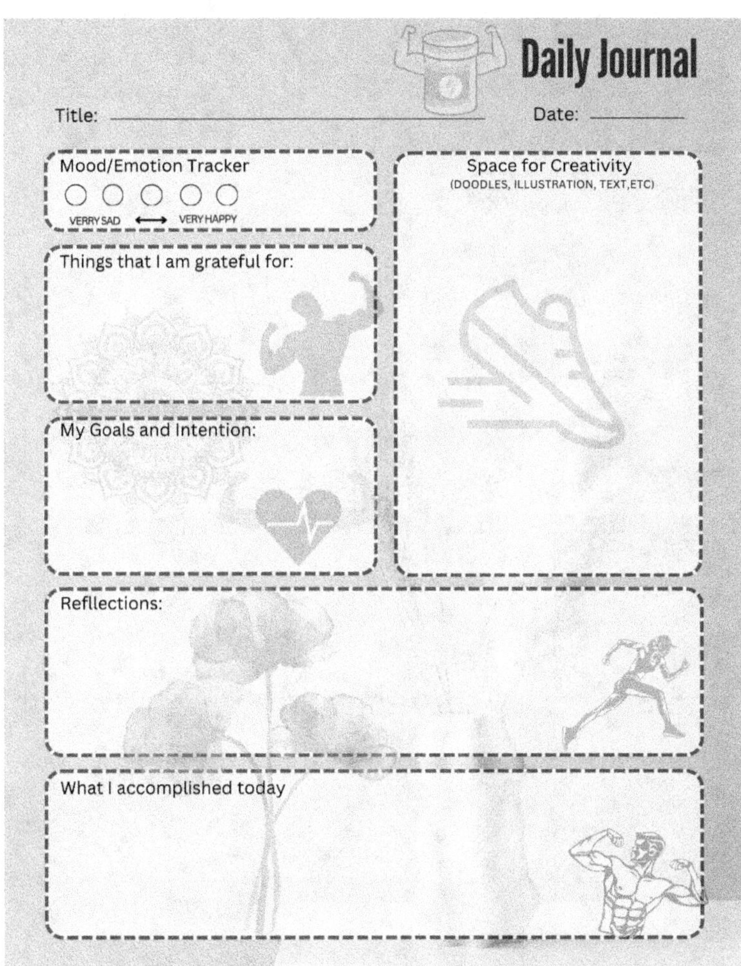

Daily Journal

Title: ___________________________   Date: ___________

Mood/Emotion Tracker

○ ○ ○ ○ ○

VERRY SAD ←→ VERY HAPPY

Things that I am grateful for:

My Goals and Intention:

Space for Creativity
(DOODLES, ILLUSTRATION, TEXT,ETC)

Refllections:

What I accomplished today

Daily Journal

Title: _______________________ Date: _______________

Mood/Emotion Tracker

○ ○ ○ ○ ○

VERRY SAD ⟷ VERY HAPPY

Things that I am grateful for:

My Goals and Intention:

Space for Creativity
(DOODLES, ILLUSTRATION, TEXT,ETC)

Refllections:

What I accomplished today

Daily Journal

Title: _______________________________ Date: ___________

Mood/Emotion Tracker

○ ○ ○ ○ ○

VERRY SAD ←——→ VERY HAPPY

Things that I am grateful for:

My Goals and Intention:

Space for Creativity
(DOODLES, ILLUSTRATION, TEXT,ETC)

Refllections:

What I accomplished today

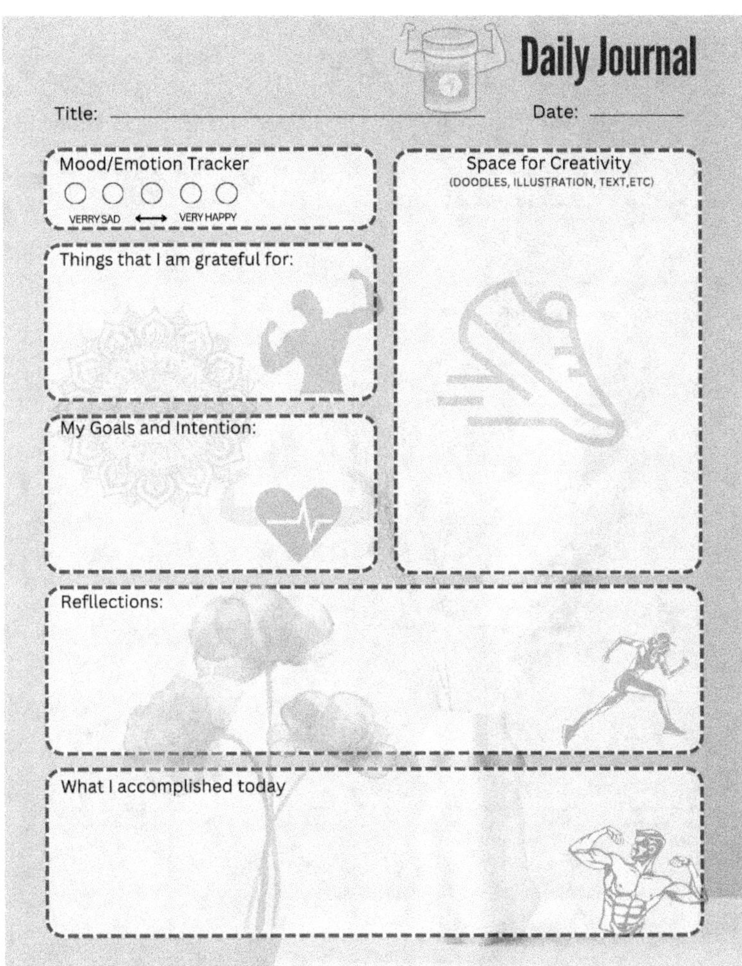

Daily Journal

Title: _______________________________   Date: __________

Mood/Emotion Tracker

◯ ◯ ◯ ◯ ◯

VERRY SAD ⟷ VERY HAPPY

Space for Creativity
(DOODLES, ILLUSTRATION, TEXT,ETC)

Things that I am grateful for:

My Goals and Intention:

Refllections:

What I accomplished today

Daily Journal

Title: _______________________   Date: _________

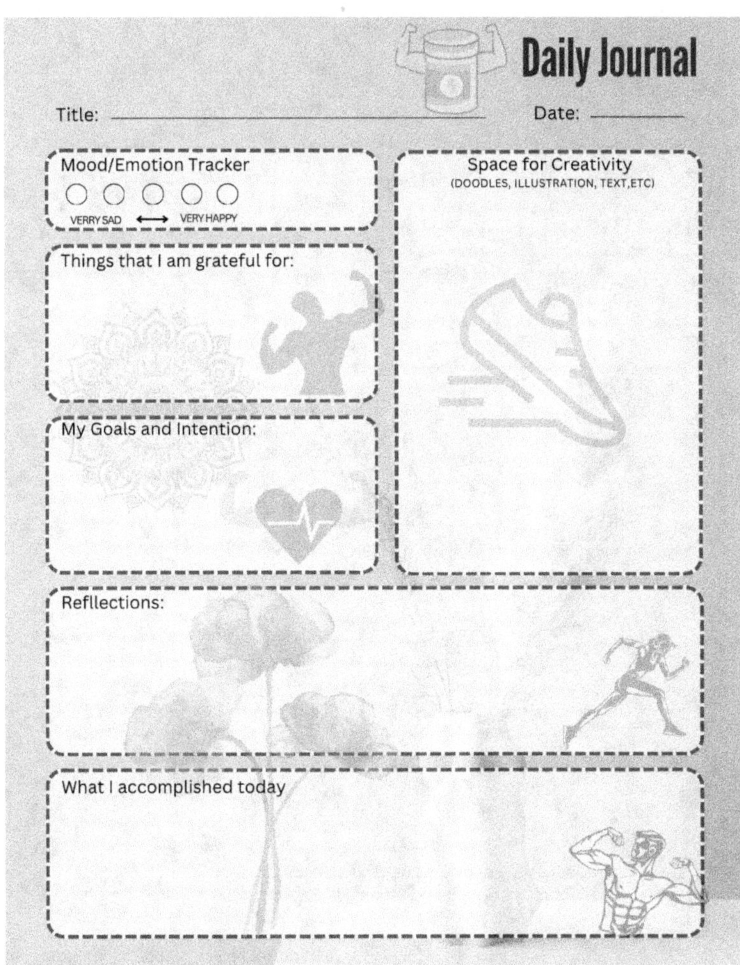

Mood/Emotion Tracker

○ ○ ○ ○ ○

VERRY SAD ←——→ VERY HAPPY

Things that I am grateful for:

My Goals and Intention:

Space for Creativity
(DOODLES, ILLUSTRATION, TEXT,ETC)

Refllections:

What I accomplished today

Daily Journal

Title: _______________________________   Date: ___________

Mood/Emotion Tracker

○ ○ ○ ○ ○

VERRY SAD ⟷ VERY HAPPY

Things that I am grateful for:

My Goals and Intention:

Space for Creativity
(DOODLES, ILLUSTRATION, TEXT,ETC)

Refllections:

What I accomplished today

Daily Journal

Title: __________________________   Date: __________

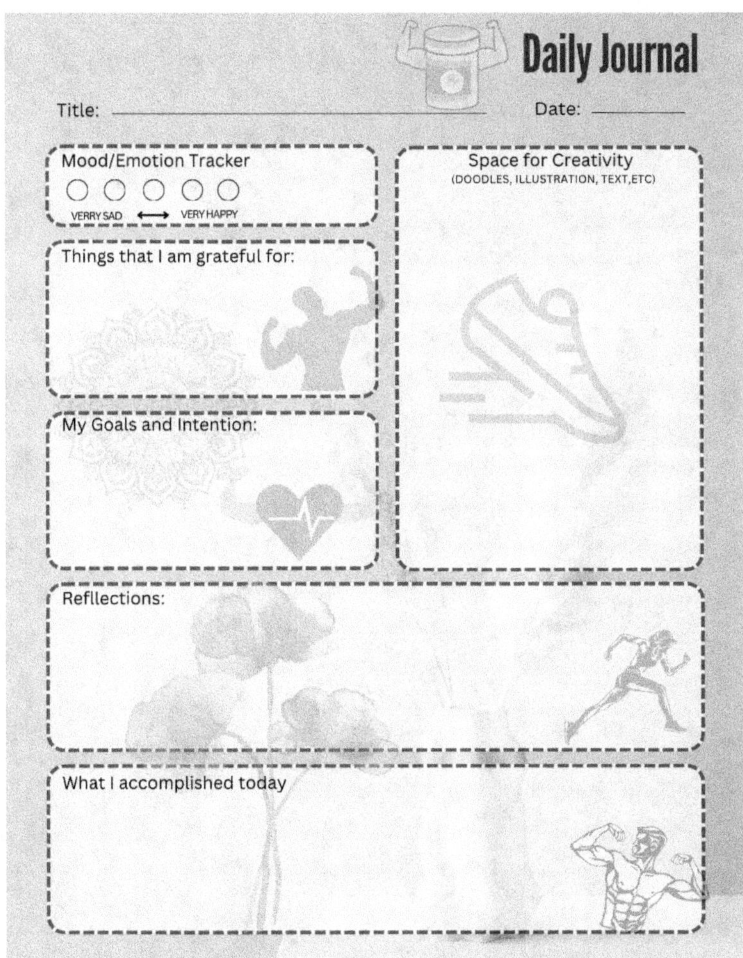

Mood/Emotion Tracker

◯ ◯ ◯ ◯ ◯

VERRY SAD ⟷ VERY HAPPY

Things that I am grateful for:

My Goals and Intention:

Space for Creativity
(DOODLES, ILLUSTRATION, TEXT,ETC)

Refllections:

What I accomplished today

Daily Journal

Title: _______________________________   Date: _________

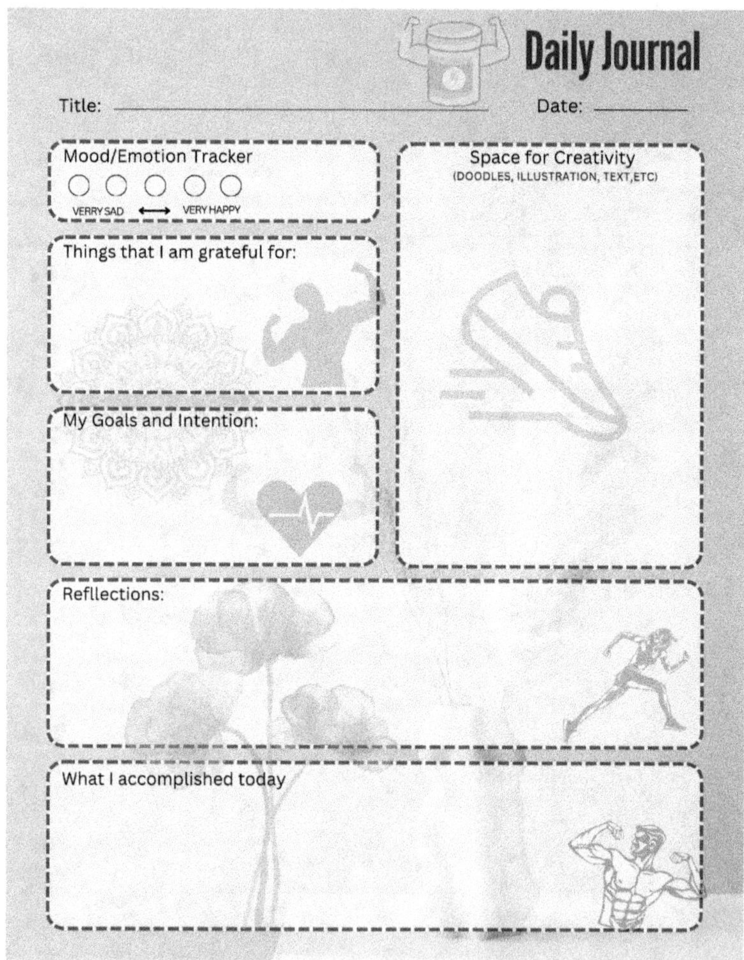

Mood/Emotion Tracker

VERRY SAD ⟷ VERY HAPPY

Things that I am grateful for:

My Goals and Intention:

Space for Creativity
(DOODLES, ILLUSTRATION, TEXT,ETC)

Refllections:

What I accomplished today

Daily Journal

Title: _______________________   Date: _______

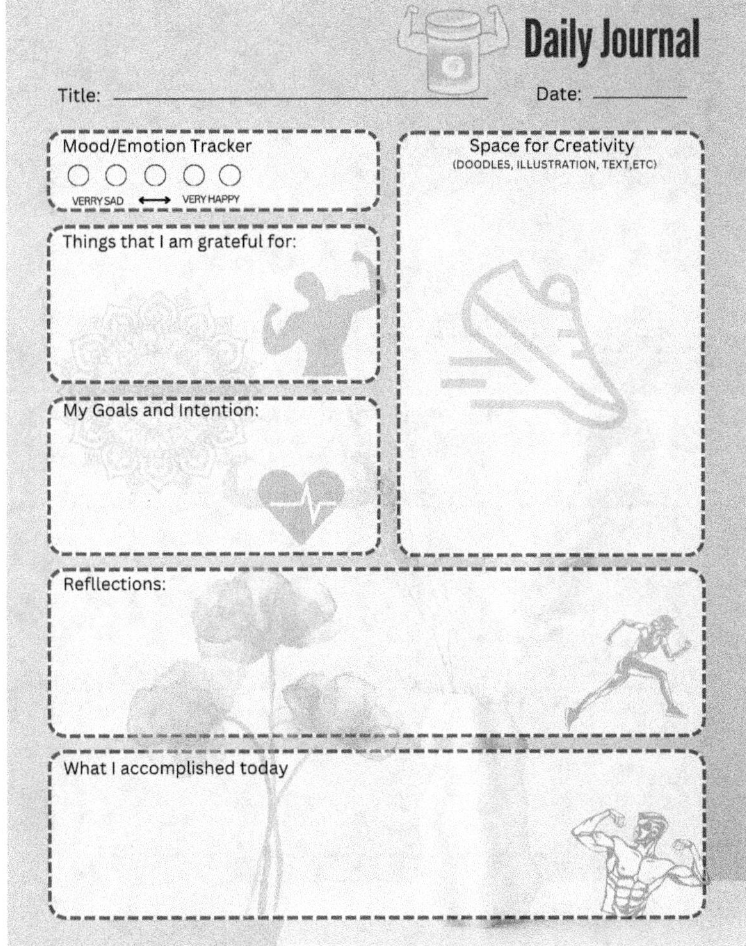

Daily Journal

Title: _______________________________   Date: _________

Mood/Emotion Tracker

○ ○ ○ ○ ○

VERRY SAD ←——→ VERY HAPPY

Things that I am grateful for:

My Goals and Intention:

Space for Creativity
(DOODLES, ILLUSTRATION, TEXT,ETC)

Refllections:

What I accomplished today

Daily Journal

Title: _______________________________   Date: _________

Things that I am grateful for:

My Goals and Intention:

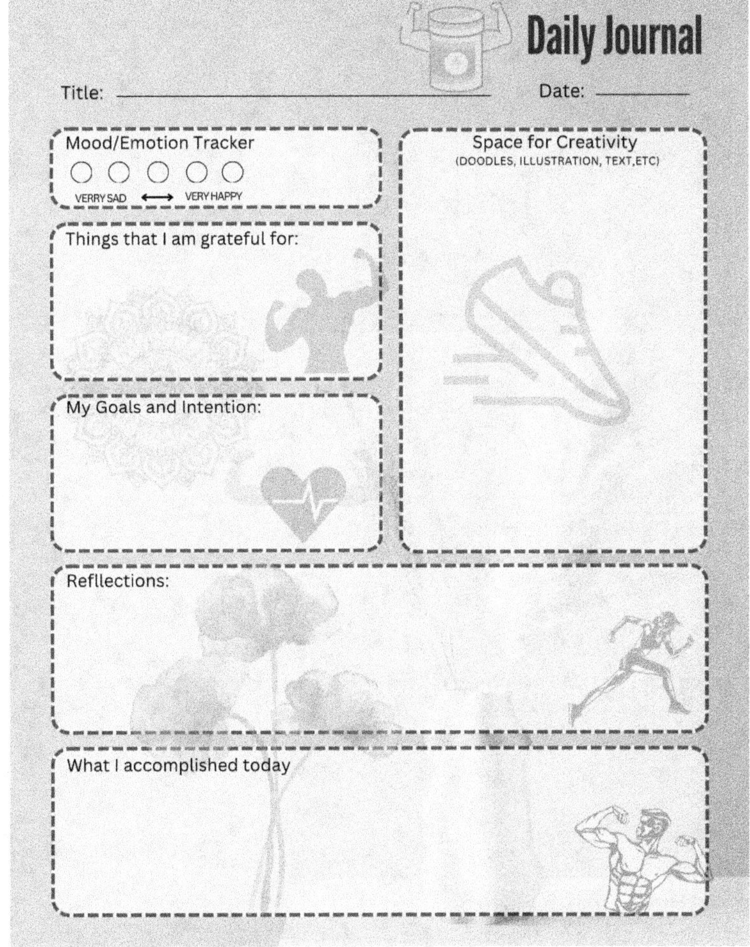

Refllections:

What I accomplished today

Daily Journal

Title: _______________________________   Date: _________

Mood/Emotion Tracker

○ ○ ○ ○ ○

VERRY SAD ⟷ VERY HAPPY

Things that I am grateful for:

My Goals and Intention:

Space for Creativity
(DOODLES, ILLUSTRATION, TEXT,ETC)

Refllections:

What I accomplished today